THE NEW ART OF LONGEVITY

HOW TO LIVE LONG AND HEALTHY

HENRY MATTHIAS

CONTENTS

INTRODUCTION

Everyone wants a long life. Advances in medicine now treat and even cure the diseases that once came with lethal prognoses. Today's medicine enables us to live long and full lives that our ancestors could not have imagined.

A century ago, an infection often resulted in death. Advances in antibiotics combat infection with greater power and efficacy than ever before. Systemic diseases like diabetes and HIV, while still deadly if left untreated, can now be managed with today's advanced medicine.

Life expectancy has increased over the past century, too. According to the BBC (Ruggeri, 2018), the average person born in 1960, which is the earliest year the

United Nations began archiving global data, could expect to live 52.5 years. Today, the average lifespan worldwide is 72 years. We have medical advances to thank for that, too.

We need not rely on advanced medicine to live a long, productive life. Any individual can live longer through the self-determined actions highlighted in this book. As you read this book, review the strategies herein—all backed by science—to help you live longer and be happier by making some simple and powerful lifestyle changes.

THE IMPORTANCE OF ROUTINE DOCTOR VISITS

Before taking any action to improve your health and live longer, you need to determine the status of your health. There's no better way to do this than to visit your physician. Do not assume you are healthy or that your aches and pains are merely an inevitable part of aging. Many diseases lurk beneath surface awareness and may be treated or rectified under the regular care of a doctor.

PROLONG YOUR LIFE WITH REGULAR DOCTOR VISITS

A physician keeps a record of your health, which enables him or her to detect subtle changes that may indicate a need for intervention. Such trends may involve regular testing of hormone levels, recording your blood pressure and weight, and more. Although you may be tempted to avoid seeing your doctor when minor aches and pains arise because you believe they will ease in time, have you considered the consequences of what may happen if those supposedly minor discomforts don't go away?

Seemingly minor issues may deepen and spread when left untreated, resulting in emergency treatment or drastic measures that could have been avoided with early detection and treatment. Failure to visit your doctor regularly means you will not know what is wrong until the problem becomes advanced or even life-threatening.

Included in regular doctor visits is a comprehensive annual checkup. For many, healthcare insurance covers the cost of this full scan of one's health, and many such policies *require* that the person insured get an annual checkup in order to maintain coverage. However, policies differ, so speak to your insurer to understand what your health insurance does and does not cover.

A comprehensive checkup often includes various scans and tests as well as physical examinations to detect the presence of disease. These include mammograms, pelvic exams, pap smears, colonoscopies, blood panels, and more. Sex, age, family history, diet, and family history all affect your health. Discuss the appropriate health scans with your physician and pay for them out-of-pocket if necessary.

DON'T RELY ON SELF-DIAGNOSIS

The internet can be an excellent source of information —and misinformation. Powerful search engines deploying artificial intelligence and websites purporting to address all types of ailments may imbue you with a false sense of competence when it comes to identifying and treating your own health problems. Many diseases have the same general symptoms; deeper analysis is needed to identify the specific health problem ailing you.

Your doctor keeps a record of data pertaining to your specific health. Although you, too, maybe monitoring your blood pressure and other vital statistics regularly, you could jeopardize your well-being by relying on a website trying to sell you a miracle cure or advocating for a home remedy. Without knowing the potency or lack thereof of the herbs or essential oils you use to formulate a home remedy, you may be doing yourself more harm than good.

If you feel unwell, see your doctor. A trained physician has a much better chance of accurately diagnosing your health problem(s) and prescribing the proper treatment than anyone without such training.

2

THE BENEFIT OF THE GREAT OUTDOORS

GETTING VITAMIN D

Scientific research proves that the great outdoors is good for you. Exposure to sunshine helps your body create vitamin D, which helps your body absorb and retain calcium and phosphorus, which are critical elements for building and maintaining strong bones. According to Harvard University, "laboratory studies show that vitamin D can reduce cancer cell growth, help control infections and reduce inflammation" (Harvard T.H. Chan School of Public Health, 2023).

Public health messages in recent decades have focused on the hazards of prolonged exposure to ultraviolet light leads to sunburn and may even cause damage to one's DNA and various skin cancers. However, you don't need to risk your health to get the benefits of sunshine. Ten to thirty minutes of daily exposure of approximately twenty-five percent of your skin to sunlight is sufficient to generate one's daily requirement of vitamin D. People with darker skin may need more prolonged exposure to get the same benefit.[1]

Beyond a healthy skeletal system, vitamin D acquired via exposure to sunshine also confers other benefits. According to the National Institutes of Health (Mead, 2008), *low* exposure to sunlight has been linked to many major illnesses, such as multiple sclerosis, type 1 and 2 diabetes, and hypertension. Adequate sun exposure may even confer protection against rheumatoid arthritis, asthma, and infectious diseases.

BEYOND VITAMIN D

In addition to the above-mentioned physical benefits, surrounding oneself with nature also confers emotional and mental benefits. According to Healthline (Swain, 2022), the benefits of spending time outdoors include the following:

- Improved respiration
- Eased or reduced depression
- Greater motivation to exercise
- Mental Restoration

- Improved immune function
- Protection from myopia
- Improved emotional well-being
- Improved sleep.

That last item leads us to the next section.

3

GET YOUR FORTY WINKS

Research has long shown that getting sufficient sleep is critical to one's good health. Getting a good night's sleep on a consistent basis "helps you recover from injuries faster and improves your overall health and resistance to illness" (Stuart Schmidt, n.d.).

It is easy to deprive yourself of enough sleep: stress, worry, work, and other reasons make relaxation difficult for many people. Lack of sleep directly affects immune function, too (Stuart Schmidt, n.d.). A good night's sleep every night is a priority. Failure to get those forty winks is detrimental to your physical and mental health and results in faster aging.

CONSISTENCY IS KEY

Consistent sleep is critical to living a longer, healthier life and greater well-being. A consistent sleep habit requires developing and maintaining routines:

- Go to bed and wake up at the same time every day.
- Refrain from spending time on your phone or computer or watching TV for at least 30 minutes before going to bed.
- Don't engage in intense exercise close to bedtime.
- Avoid caffeinated beverages late in the day.

The correct amount of sleep one needs depends on the individual. As a rule, children require more sleep—around ten hours each night—than adults, who need a *minimum* of six hours nightly.

THE LINK BETWEEN SLEEP AND LONGEVITY

Studies confirm that lack of sleep increases one's risk of early death by as much as twelve percent. During slumber, your body heals, repairing damaged cells. Poor or insufficient sleep leads to obesity, diabetes, and heart disease, which all contribute to a shortened lifespan.

However, getting too much sleep is not good either. An occasional nap doesn't mean you're getting too much sleep. Oversleeping may be caused by excessive alcohol consumption, certain prescription medications, stress, worry, and other issues.

Those who suffer from excess sleep or hypersomnia experience symptoms of anxiety, lethargy, and memory problems. Too much sleep also contributes to obesity, headaches, back pain, depression, and heart disease. Adults who consistently sleep nine or more hours a night have significantly higher death rates than those who consistently sleep seven to eight hours per night.[1]

YOU ARE SUPERMAN!

"What is a superhero? They're supposed to represent hope, opportunity, and strength for everybody."

— ALDIS HODGE

Well, okay, perhaps you're not Superman, and no matter how much you improve your health and well-being, you'll never be immortal... But there's still a parallel to be drawn here... Stay with me...

Superman draws his power from the sun – it's not a given. If he were to keep himself away from the sun for an extended period, his powers would wane. The tools and strategies you're learning here are akin to Superman's sun – avoid implementing them, and you're going to risk your chances of living a long and healthy life.

We all want to be Superman. We all want to live for as long as we can in the best shape possible. And while there's no chance of acquiring superpowers, there are things we can do to cultivate and maintain the powers we already have.

When you implement the strategies in this book, you're putting yourself in control of your health and longevity – you're maintaining your power and making sure you're just about as much of a superhero as it's possible for a human being to be.

My goal with this book is to help as many people as I can to live a long and productive life – simply by making lifestyle changes… and you can help me.

By leaving a review of this book on Amazon, you'll show new readers where they can find exactly the guidance they need to supercharge their health and follow the path to a long and happy life.

Simply by telling other readers how this book has helped you and what they'll find inside, you'll channel your inner Superman (or Superwoman) and help someone else find the power within them.

Thank you so much for your support. Life expectancy is increasing – let's make sure as many of us as possible get to enjoy that for all it's worth.

4

YOU ARE WHAT YOU EAT: THE IMPORTANCE OF DIET

A proper diet is crucial to living a longer, healthier life. It is said that if you don't treat food as medicine, then medicine will become your food.

Three factors of your diet directly impact your lifespan and are related to obesity, antioxidants, and cholesterol. Arranging your diet to avoid obesity, increasing the amount of antioxidants you consume, and minimizing "bad" cholesterol and saturated fats does not necessarily require drastic changes in what you eat. In other words, you need not convert to any radical dietary practice.

Antioxidants prevent or delay cell damage by counteracting oxidative stress and are found in the diet of fruits and vegetables. Evidence shows that antioxidants may help prevent chronic ailments, such as cardiovascular diseases, cancer, and cataracts; however, they may also interact with some medications. A diet rich in fruit and vegetables will supply the necessary antioxidants your body needs.[1]

Low-density lipoprotein (LDL) cholesterol, also called "bad" cholesterol, raises one's risk for heart disease and stroke. It collects in the walls of blood vessels and blocks them.[2] Your liver makes its own LDL cholesterol; the food you eat adds to that. High LDL levels indicate high triglycerides, meaning an excess of fat, and lead to heart problems.

Foods that lower LDL cholesterol include almonds, orange juice, olive oil, steamed vegetables (e.g., asparagus, okra, carrots, beets, green beans, eggplant, cauliflower), oatmeal, pinto beans, blueberries, tomatoes, avocados, dark chocolate (70 percent cacao minimum), barley, pectin-rich fruits (e.g., pears, apples, plums), soy (i.e., tofu), and omega-3 fatty fish (e.g., salmon, tuna, trout).

Obesity refers to a body mass index (BMI) over 30, a level of excessive weight that negatively affects every aspect of health: reproductive, respiratory, cardiovascular, muscular, skeletal, mental well-being, mood, and more. It increases the risk of debilitating and deadly diseases such as heart disease, diabetes, and cancer.

Foods that support a healthy weight loss program include whole eggs, leafy greens, salmon, cruciferous vegetables (e.g., broccoli, cabbage), chicken breast and lean meats, potatoes, and other root vegetables *without the butter, cheese, and sour cream* (e.g., turnips, parsnips, beets), tuna, and legumes (e.g., lentils, black beans, kidney beans). Regular exercise also supports weight loss.

Likely, you already know what foods are good for you and what is not. It's probable you already know which certain foods are considered "junk food" or are regarded as treats to be consumed on an occasional basis. This means consuming less refined sugars (including sucrose, fructose, corn syrup, etc.), fewer saturated fats, and fewer carbohydrates (starches, processed grains). A healthful diet consists of fresh fruit and vegetables, lean meats and fish, and plenty of water.

CHANGE YOUR DIET, CHANGE YOUR LIFESTYLE

A successful transition from an unhealthy diet to a healthy one requires commitment and the mindful consumption of food and beverages. Switch from snacking on junk food (e.g., candy bars, potato chips) to raw vegetables or fresh fruit. Drink water instead of sugar-laden soft drinks. Avoid heavy sauces made with lots of cream, butter, or cheese. Reduce the amount of salt you use when cooking and seasoning your food. Opt for whole-grain bread and brown rice rather than refined wheat or white rice. Resist processed meats like sausage and bologna, which are filled with salt and fat.

In addition to adjusting what you eat, it is also important to **control the size of the portions you eat**. It is a truism that if you are served larger portions of food, then you will eat more. Doubling portion size leads to an average 35 percent increase in consumption (Holden, 2014). This may arise from conditioning by one's parents to "clean your plate," a habit of consuming a fixed portion of whatever is served, or other failures of internal awareness when enough is enough.

To control your portion size, first, begin with a smaller plate. Then divide your plate into quarters. Two of the four quarters (or half of the plate) should be filled with fresh vegetables or fruit. Fill one-quarter with starchy food such as potatoes, bread, or pasta. Fill the final portion with protein (e.g., meat).

CONSIDER INTERMITTENT FASTING

Most diets result in weight loss by reducing one's consumption of total daily calories. The latest weight loss trend, **intermittent fasting**, builds on this with the theory that this type of diet decreases appetite by slowing the body's metabolism (William Kormos, 2017). Studies show that intermittent fasting works. "A 2020 review that included 27 IF trials found that the programs led to a weight loss of 0.8 percent to 13.0 percent of baseline weight without serious side effects in every study" (Abbey Sharp, 2020).

Although it has become a recent trend, fasting as a dietary practice is ancient. It involves alternating cycles of abstention from food and/or drink. Most intermittent fasting practices do not dictate what foods or how much one should consume during the periods of scheduled consumption. Regardless of the period, intermittent fasting allows for drinking noncaloric beverages (e.g., water, plain tea, or coffee) anytime.

Intermittent fasting comes in an array of standard methods denoted by the hours of abstention and the hours of consumption. Extreme fasting practices restrict food consumption to alternate days rather than cycles within the same 24-hour period.

The benefit of intermittent fasting is weight management, assuming one refrain from gorging during the consumption period. Weight management or weight loss generally comes from eating proper proportions of a healthful diet, meaning one eats less overall. Intermittent fasting improves mental acuity by preventing short-term and special memory loss and reducing brain damage and functional impairment. It has been shown to help people control their blood sugar and to reduce visceral belly fat, fasting insulin, and insulin resistance. For those undergoing chemo-therapy, intermittent fasting shows promise as a tool to minimize the side effects of treatment and boost the treatment's efficacy.

If you decide to participate in intermittent fasting, be aware of its drawbacks. It can impair athletic perfor-mance, depriving your body of the fuel it needs when it needs it. It is difficult to maintain, especially the more radical methods. It may contribute to binging. The long-term effects of intermittent fasting are unknown.[3]

DRINK WATER FOR LONGEVITY

Sweet soft drinks inundate the body with lots of empty calories if made with sugar (e.g., cane sugar, corn syrup, dextrose, fructose) and, especially with artificially sweetened beverages, lots of addictive chemicals. Beverages containing sugar not only promote tooth decay but also contribute to unhealthy weight gain, high blood sugar, high blood pressure, inflammation, obesity, and atherosclerosis—all of which are factors for heart disease. If you think that ingesting food or beverages loaded with artificial sweeteners will avoid those problems, think again. Side effects of artificial sweeteners (e.g., sugar alcohols, stevia, luo han guo) encompass intestinal issues, increased blood sugar, bladder cancer, high blood pressure, headache, brain tumors, increased appetite, and even adverse effects on pre-existing mood disorders.

The solution is to **drink water**. Water comprises around 60 percent of the human body, so it's important to stay hydrated. Staying hydrated supports physical performance prevents headaches and constipation, and more. Losing as little as 2 percent of one's body's water content can significantly impair physical performance. Dehydration negatively affects the body's ability to control its temperature. It leads to a decrease in motivation and an increase in fatigue.

Brain function and health also depend upon proper hydration. Losing as little as 1 to 3 percent of your body's water content results in headaches, a decrease in working memory, and increased fatigue and anxiety. Dehydration also causes headaches and, in some people, migraines. Proper hydration also relieves hangovers.

Low water consumption leads to intestinal issues like constipation and other painful problems such as kidney stones. Although a higher fluid intake increases urine output, it also keeps the kidneys flushed and dilutes the concentration of minerals, thereby preventing kidney disease and kidney stones.

Water not only fills the stomach, thereby decreasing hunger and the urge to snack, but it can also boost one's metabolic rate. Timing is important when drinking water as a part of a weight loss program. Drinking water half an hour before meals hastens feelings of satiation, so you eat less.

5

EXERCISE YOUR BODY ... AND YOUR BRAIN

Research confirms what we already know: a sedentary lifestyle leads to a shortened lifespan. The amount of muscle mass one has indicates one's longevity. As adults age, we gradually lose muscle mass, strength, and function. This condition involving muscle atrophy, called sarcopenia, affects the musculoskeletal system and factors in increased frailty, falls, and bone fractures which may lead to hospitalization and death. Symptoms of sarcopenia include loss of stamina, poor balance, and weakness.

INCREASE MUSCLE MASS AND LONGEVITY WITH EXERCISE

Regular exercise helps to maintain or even increase muscle mass as well as enables your body to manufacture more stem cells. Stem cells adapt to your body's needs, becoming the types of cells the body requires as they are required. The increase in stem cell production enables the body to replace worn or dead cells throughout the body more regularly, thereby engaging in a perpetual system of renewal. Because of this, a consistent exercise regimen leads to the growth of more muscle cells, thereby increasing one's muscle mass.

Enjoying the benefits of youthful renewal through exercise does not require grueling rigor or countless hours of sweaty exertion; however, it does require a commitment to exercise every day. Establish a modest routine of thirty minutes daily. Begin slowly with a low-intensity activity so as not to overstrain your body and injure yourself, then gradually increase both the effort and the length of time. The results will come—not immediately—in the form of greater strength, better balance, stronger mental acuity, more agility, improved stamina, and a host of other mental and physical benefits.

EXERCISE YOUR BRAIN, TOO

Beyond the benefits of physical exercise, mental exercise helps keep the mind sharp and the brain functioning at peak capacity. To exercise the brain, learn something new. Challenge your thinking and perceptions. Embark upon new experiences and develop new skills.

Mental exercises, new experiences, and engaged learning work the brain's "muscles," strengthening them and making the mind more limber and resilient. These activities, which include solving puzzles and reading, build new neural pathways and help the brain to function better.

6

THE IMPORTANCE OF SOCIALIZING

If the COVID-19 pandemic and the lockdown strictures imposed upon communities worldwide taught us anything, it is that **loneliness is lethal**. Humanity being a social species, longevity requires community and a network for social interaction and support. Science proves that people who are better connected with family members and friends tend to be healthier than those who live in social isolation. Physical, mental, and emotional well-being requires human interaction.

HEALTH RISKS OF LONELINESS

Especially for the elderly, evidence shows that social isolation and loneliness, although impossible to precisely quantify, increase a person's risk by 50 percent of premature death from *all* causes. In short, loneliness is a greater risk to longevity than air pollution, obesity, smoking, and alcohol abuse. According to the Centers for Disease Control (Centers for Disease Control 2021), social isolation was associated with about a 50 percent increased risk of dementia, a 29 percent increased risk of heart disease, a 32 percent increased risk of stroke, and higher rates of depression, anxiety, and suicide. Chronic loneliness affects everything, from poor diet to sleep deprivation to chronic inflammation.

BENEFITS OF SOCIAL CONNECTION

Not only is socializing with friends and family fun, but it is also good for your mind and body. Socializing combats loneliness, if only because the brain can relax from a state of hypervigilance required to survive. In short, it is a herd mentality that relies upon the communal nature of the herd to detect danger and alert others to its presence: there is safety in numbers. Socializing also helps sharpen memory, improves mental acuity, improves hormonal activity, increases one's sense of well-being, and is thought to help you live longer.

COMMUNITY REQUIRES COMMUNICATION

Of course, building and maintaining a positive social circle requires a bit of effort and even some skill. To stave off loneliness and reap the benefits of positive social engagement, you must demonstrate good communication skills. Improving the way you communicate with others strengthens your connections with them.

Real communication in relationships builds trust, improves conflict resolution, and increases intimacy. The core aspect of a strong social connection is a true connection. This true connection is not relegated to small talk but engages verbal, physical, and written skills to support the other person and fulfill his or her needs. It requires understanding—although not necessarily agreeing with—different viewpoints and inspiring others to reciprocate.

You can do this by supporting others. Studies show that people who support others tend to be healthier and have longer lifespans. Supporting others gains you personal satisfaction and deepens the relationship you have with those whom you support. In return, they are more likely to support you when you need it.

Motivational speaker Tony Robbins identifies four basic communication styles: passive, aggressive, passive-aggressive, and assertive. Of the four, the healthiest type of communication is assertive because assertive people are in touch with their emotions and know how to communicate them effectively (Tony Robbins, n.d.). Positive communication does not mean slathering compliments; it refers to tact and honesty, an ability to let go of grudges and break negative patterns, and a willingness to start over.

CONCLUSION

Genetic predisposition and catastrophic events aside, you have the power to increase your life span. You control your lifestyle, your diet, and your social connections—all the things that affect your health, well-being, and longevity.

One of the most important factors in prolonging your life is happiness. Happiness here does not refer to an ephemeral pleasure or moment of joy but to a consistently positive mindset. This takes commitment and requires avoidance or adroit handling of negative emotions and reducing stress. Optimists live up to 15 percent longer than pessimists, according to a study spanning thousands of people and three decades (Lewina O. Lee 2019). While the study did not conclude any specific reasons for the health and longevity benefits of optimism, it suggests that an optimistic mindset leads to healthy behaviors and helps people avoid unhealthy impulses. Optimists may also cope better with stress and enabling them to pursue long-term rewards rather than instant gratification in challenging situations.

If you are a pessimist or a cynical realist, then changing your mindset is possible, if not necessarily easy. To change your brain from pessimism to optimism, practice gratitude, acknowledge other possibilities, rephrase your words, acknowledge your empowerment, find the silver lining, focus on the present, control your thoughts, and find a mentor.

Remember to relax your mind and body. Relaxation relieves stress and its harmful side effects, as well as helps you get in touch with yourself. Do this through prayer, mindful meditation, or other practices. Listening to music can help, too. Learn to breathe deeply and clear your mind and regain your focus to improve and prolong your life.

NOTES

2. THE BENEFIT OF THE GREAT OUTDOORS

1. Lizzie Streit, MS, RDN, LD., Vitamins C and D: What You Need To Know, August 4, 2021, https://sogoodsoyou.com/blogs/news/vitamins-c-and-d

3. GET YOUR FORTY WINKS

1. Krishnan SSG, Too much of anything is fit for nothing, July 2022, https://reflections.live/articles/1347/too-much-of-anything-is-fit-for-nothing-an-article-by-krishnan-ssg-5581-l64uk5yu.html

4. YOU ARE WHAT YOU EAT: THE IMPORTANCE OF DIET

1. 6 THINGS YOU NEED TO KNOW ABOUT MOUTH CANCER, 16th October 2018, https://www.cgdp.com/2018/10/16/6-things-you-need-to-know-about-mouth-cancer/
2. Rare Gene Found Among Amish Populations Help Protect Against Heart Disease, Tuesday, December 21, 2021, https://www.punnettssquare.com/2021/12/rare-gene-found-among-amish-populations.html
3. What to know about the monk fast, https://www.medicalnewstoday.com/articles/monk-fast

REFERENCES

Abbey Sharp, RD. 2020. *Want to Try Intermittent Fasting? Here's What You Need to Know.* October 7. Accessed May 22, 2023. https://greatist.com/eat/intermittent-fasting-health-benefits-and-side-effects.

Centers for Disease Control. 2021. *Loneliness and Social Isolation Linked to Serious Health Conditions.* April 29. Accessed May 22, 2023. https://www.cdc.gov/aging/publications/features/lonely-older-adults.html.

Harvard T.H. Chan School of Public Health. 2023. *The Nutrition Source.* March. Accessed May 22, 2023. https://www.hsph.harvard.edu/nutritionsource/vitamin-d/.

Holden, Stephen S. 2014. *Health Check: Do Bigger Portion Sizes Make You Eat More?* April 14. Accessed May 22, 2023. https://www.theepochtimes.com/health/health-check-do-bigger-portion-sizes-make-you-eat-more_620729.html.

Lewina O. Lee, Peter James, Emily S. Zevon, Eric S. Kim, Claudia Trudel-Fitzgerald, Avron Spiro III, Francine Grodstein, and Laura D. Kubzansky. 2019. *Optimism Is Associated with Exceptional Longevity in 2 Epidemiologic Cohorts of Men and Women.* August 26. Accessed May 22, 2023. https://www.pnas.org/doi/full/10.1073/pnas.1900712116.

Lil Tigers. (2023, April 24). *85 Best Superhero Quotes To Inspire & Motivate.* https://liltigers.net/superhero-quotes-for-kids/

Mead, N. Nathaniel. 2008. *Benefits of Sunlight.* April 11. Accessed May 22, 2023. https://www.ncbi.nlm.nih.gov/pmc/articles/PMC2290997/.

Ruggeri, Amanda. 2018. *100 Year Life.* October 2. Accessed May 22, 2023. https://www.bbc.com/future/article/20181002-how-long-did-ancient-people-live-life-span-versus-longevity.

Stuart Schmidt, MS, ATC, CSCS. n.d. *Sleep for Health and*

Performance. Accessed May 22, 2023. https://www.centerfounda tion.org/sleep-for-health/.

Swain, Emily. 2022. *8 Health Benefits of Getting Back to Nature and Spending Time Outside.* May 28. Accessed May 22, 2023. https:// www.healthline.com/health/health-benefits-of-being-outdoors.

Tony Robbins. n.d. *How to Communicate in a Relationship.* Accessed May 22, 2023. https://www.tonyrobbins.com/ultimate-relationship-guide/key-communication-relationships/.

William Kormos, MD. 2017. *Any Benefits to Intermittent Fasting?* January 13. Accessed May 22, 2023. https://www.health.harvard.edu/diet-and-weight-loss/any-benefits-to-intermittent-fasting-diets.

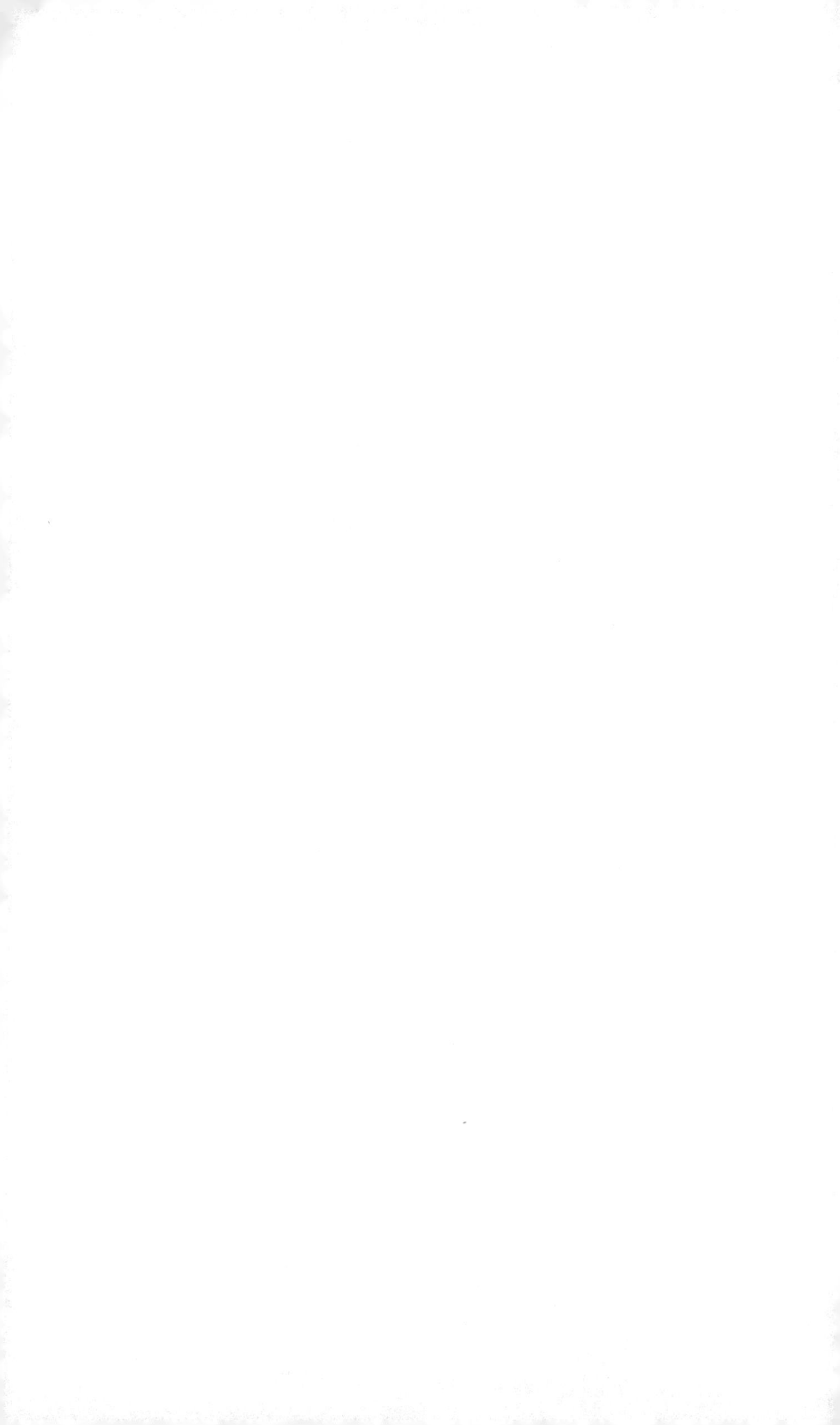

www.ingramcontent.com/pod-product-compliance
Lightning Source LLC
Chambersburg PA
CBHW051401250726
48656CB00006B/2203